Charcot Marie Tooth Disease

Diagnosis, Symptoms, Treatment, Causes,
Doctors, Nervous Disorders, Prognosis, Research,
History, Surgery, and More!

By Frederick Earlstein

Copyrights and Trademarks

Disclaimer and Legal Notice

Foreword

Charcot Marie Tooth disease is one of the most common inherited neurological conditions in existence, affecting approximately 1 in 2,500 people – that equates to more than 26,000 people in the United Kingdom and nearly 130,000 people in the United States. The causes of this disease are still being studied and, unfortunately, there is no standard treatment. Charcot Marie Tooth disease comes in several different forms with symptoms presenting as early as childhood and adolescence or as late as middle-age.

If you or a loved one has Charcot Marie Tooth disease, the best thing you can do is arm yourself with as much knowledge about the disorder as possible. In this book you will receive a wealth of knowledge about this horrible condition including its history, signs and symptoms, causes, treatment options, and more. You will also receive valuable information about current research being conducted and background on other types of nervous disorders. While you may not be able to cure Charcot Marie Tooth disease, you can use this book as a tool to better understand it.

Table of Contents

Introduction

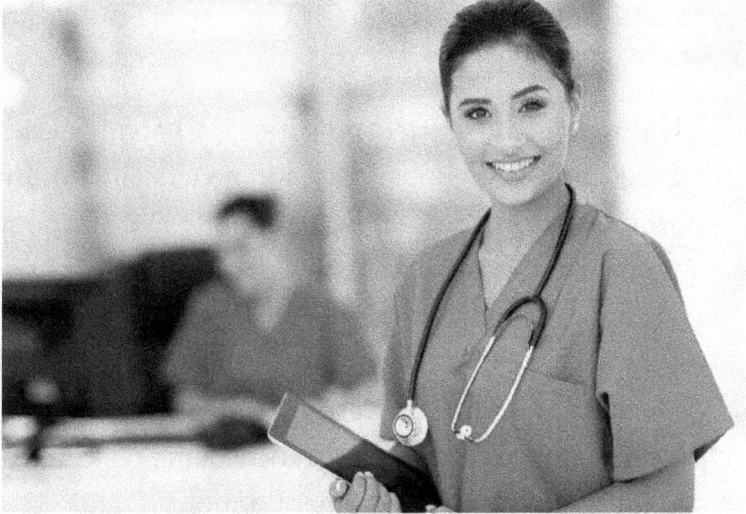

Charcot Marie Tooth disease, also known as hereditary motor and sensory neuropathy (HMSN) or peroneal muscular atrophy (PMA), is a type of inherited condition that affects the peripheral nervous system. This disease, often shortened to CMT, causes progressive muscle atrophy and loss of sensation in various parts of the body. The rate of muscle loss varies from one case to another with symptoms typically presenting in early childhood or adolescence. In some cases, however, symptoms do not present until the victim is in his or her thirties.

There is still a great deal of research being conducted regarding the cause for this disease, but it is generally accepted that genetic mutations affecting neuronal proteins are at least partially to blame. In many cases, (up to 80% of recorded cases), the primary cause of the disease is related to the duplication of part of the 17th chromosome including the gene PMP22.

Unfortunately, there is no cure for Charcot Marie Tooth disease. CMT is the most common genetically inherited neurological disorder, affecting about 1 in 2,500 people. Diagnosis of this terrible disease requires a battery of tests, not only to diagnose the condition but also to identify the type or subtype. Treatment options vary depending on the type and there is no standard treatment currently in use. Multiple clinical trials are currently being conducted to test the efficacy of various treatment options.

If you or a loved one has been diagnosed with Charcot Marie Tooth disease, you may be feeling hopeless or overwhelmed. CMT is a horrible disease – there is no doubt of that – but it can be managed and certain therapies have been shown to delay the progression. Your best weapon against Charcot Marie Tooth disease is knowledge and that is where this book comes in. Within the pages of this book you will learn everything you need to know about CMT including its history, causes, symptoms, types, treatment options, and more. By the time you finish this book you will have a thorough understanding of this condition and you will have a better idea how to treat it.

Important Terms to Know

Autosomal – A pattern of inheritance that occurs on some other type of chromosome than the X or Y.

Autosomal Dominant – A pattern of inheritance that occurs when a single copy of the mutated gene is enough to cause the disease – if a person inherits a mutated gene from their parent, both of them will have the disease.

Autosomal Recessive - A pattern of inheritance that requires two copies of the mutate gene to cause the disease. The person would receive one copy of the mutated gene from each parent and, in most cases, neither of the parents have actually developed the disease.

Axon – The gene for certain types of protein which carry electrical signals between the spinal cord and brain to the rest of the body.

Chromosome – The thread-like structures which are located in the nucleus of cells; each one is made up of protein and a single molecule of DNA.

Congenital – Present from birth; also, hereditary or inherited.

Contracture – A shortening or hardening of the muscles, tendons, or other tissues that leads to a deformity and/or rigidity of the affected joint.

Defect – An imperfection or malformation.

Foot Drop – A type of gait abnormality in which the forefoot drops due to weakness or damage of the fibular nerve; may result in difficulty lifting the foot.

Hammertoe – A bending of one or both joints in the second, third, fourth, and fifth toes, causing them to be permanently bent or curled.

Mutation – A permanent alteration of the DNA or other genetic elements.

Myelin Sheath – The protective coating around the core of a nerve fiber or axon; facilitates the transmission of nerve impulses.

Neuropathy – A term describing a problem with the nerves. Example: peripheral neuropathy.

Nerve – A single or bundle of fibers that transmits electrical impulses between the brain/spinal cord and the rest of the body.

Chapter One: What is Charcot Marie Tooth Disease?

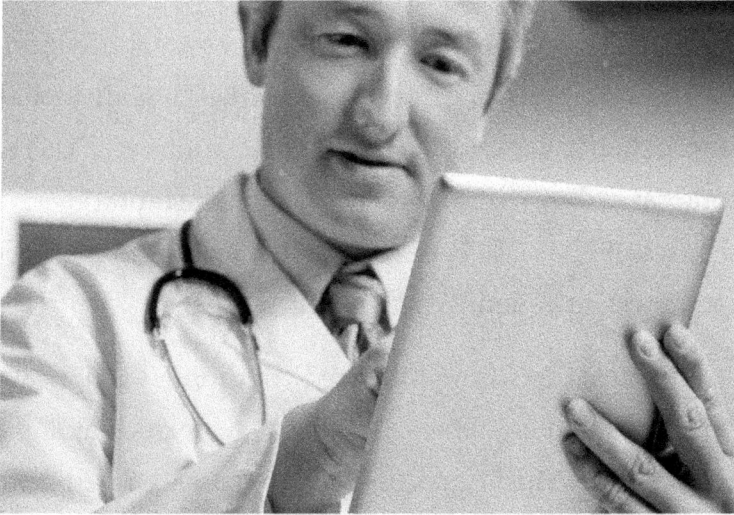

Given the name, you might assume that Charcot Marie Tooth disease is some type of periodontal disorder. In reality, however, it has nothing to do with the teeth – it is actually a type of neurological disorder affecting the peripheral nervous system. Often shortened to CMT, Charcot Marie Tooth disease is a very serious condition and it is more common than you might realize. In this chapter you will learn the basics about CMT including what it is, its history, and how it fits into the spectrum with other common nervous disorders.

1. *The Basics of Charcot Marie Tooth Disease*

The name Charcot Marie Tooth disease is applied to a group of inherited conditions that affect the peripheral nervous system. The peripheral nerves are those located outside the brain and the spinal cord. There are actually more than seventy different manifestations of CMT, each one caused by a different type of genetic mutation. New causes of CMT are being discovered each and every year as advances in genetic research are made.

Because CMT is an inherited condition it is not caused by any environmental factors – this also means that it is not contagious. Most types of CMT are passed down from one generation to the next – this is an example of dominant inheritance. Some types of the disease, however, are recessively inherited – this means that someone can have CMT even if their parents do not. In cases like this, both parents usually have a mutation in one of the two copies of the CMT gene that they carry which results in the child having two copies of the mutated gene. In rare cases, it is possible for spontaneous mutation to occur – this can happen even if neither parent has the disease.

Charcot Marie Tooth disease is the most common genetically inherited peripheral nerve disorder. This disease causes damage to the nerves that carry important signals from the brain and spinal cord to the muscles – they are also responsible for relay sensations including touch and pain. In many cases, CMT causes weakness and atrophy in the muscles as well as some loss of sensation in the hands, forearms, lower legs, and feet. Due to the abnormal tightening of muscles and the surrounding tissues, CMT can also lead to contracture, or stiff joints.

Though there are many specific causes for the different types of CMT, the general cause is a genetic defect. This defect affects the genes for certain types of protein which carry electrical signals between the spinal cord and brain to the rest of the body (called axons). It can also affect the proteins that regulate myelin, the coating on the axons. Specific genetic mutations are linked to specific types of CMT and there are more than 70 types that have been identified by researchers.

The onset and manifestation of CMT can vary depending on the type. Some cases manifest as early as birth or the disease can remain dormant until adolescence, adulthood, or late adulthood. The progression of the disease is fairly slow and it can cause different symptoms in different people. For the most part, CMT is not a life-threatening condition because it rarely affects the brain. It can, however, affect the nerves running between the diaphragm and the intercostal muscles which, in some cases, can result in respiratory impairment. There is still a great deal of research to be completed regarding the causes and types of the disease and there are several ongoing clinical trials testing different forms of treatment.

2. History of Charcot Marie Tooth Disease

Charcot Marie Tooth disease is named after not one but three physicians who were the first to describe the condition in 1886. These three physicians were Jean-Martin Charcot, Pierre Marie, and Howard Henry Tooth. The first description of the disease was published by French Professor Jean Martin Charcot (1825 – 1893) and his student, Pierre Marie (1853 – 1940). These two physicians called the disease peroneal muscular atrophy because it caused distal muscle weakness and wasting of the muscles, starting in the lower legs.

In 1886, English physician Howard Henry Tooth (1856 – 1926) described the same disease in his dissertation at Cambridge University. He called the disease peroneal progressive muscular atrophy. Though he was not the first to describe the disease, Tooth was the first to accurately attribute the symptoms to neuropathy instead of myelopathy as his predecessors had done. In 1912, another physician by the name of Hoffman described a case of peroneal muscular atrophy accompanied by thickened nerves – this disease was first named Hoffman disease but was later renamed Charcot-Marie-Tooth-Hoffman disease.

Charcot Marie Tooth disease was divided into two subtypes in 1968 – these were called CMT 1 and CMT 2. The two types were originally differentiated based on certain pathologic and physiologic criteria but later were subdivided even further based on the genetic cause of the disease. It has been hypothesized that, with developments in genetic testing, all of the different types of CMT will eventually be distinguished from one another on the basis of their genetic causes.

3. Other Common Nervous Disorders

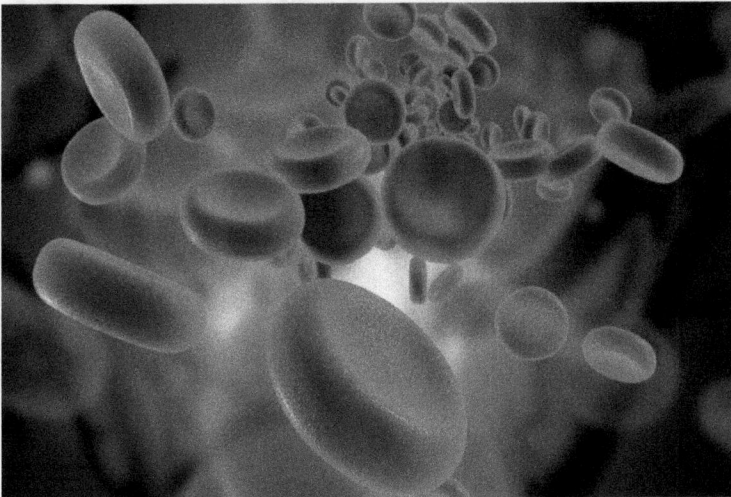

The human nervous system is a complex system that coordinates and regulates the activity of the body. There are two main divisions of the nervous system – the central nervous system and the peripheral nervous system. The central nervous system consists of the brain and spinal cord while the peripheral nervous system consists of all of the other neural elements such as the autonomic nerves and the peripheral nerves.

The nervous system controls all of your senses including sight, taste, smell, hearing and feeling. It also controls both your voluntary and involuntary functions like coordination, balance, and movement. The human nervous system controls your ability to think and to reason – it is what allows you to have memories, thoughts, and to communicate with language. The nervous system also plays a role in regulating most of the other body systems.

When it comes to disorders of the nervous system, there are a number of general categories which include:

- Infections
- Structural defects
- Vascular disorders
- Functional disorders
- Degeneration

Common infections that are likely to affect the nervous system include polio, encephalitis, meningitis and epidural abscess. The nervous system plays a role in controlling blood flow and blood pressure, so it can be affected by various vascular disorders including stroke, subdural hematoma or hemorrhage, transient ischemic attack (TIA), and subarachnoid hemorrhage. In terms of functional disorders, things like headaches, dizziness, neuralgia, and epilepsy fall into this category.

In addition to these conditions, nervous disorders can also have a serious impact on the function of the brain – especially in degenerative neurological of muscular disorders like Parkinson's and Alzheimer's disease. Other examples include multiple sclerosis, Huntington's disease, and amyotrophic lateral sclerosis (ALS). Structural disorders of the nervous system may include brain and spinal cord injuries, carpal tunnel syndrome, Bell's palsy, peripheral neuropathy, and cervical spondylosis.

Different nervous system disorders manifest in different ways, but there are some signs and symptoms that are common to many different disorders. <u>Some of the most common signs of nervous disorders include</u>:

- Persistent or sudden headaches
- Loss of feeling in the extremities
- Radiating back pain

- Weakness or loss of muscle strength
- Memory loss or impaired cognitive ability
- Loss of or change in vision
- Lack of coordination or muscle rigidity
- Tremors and/or seizures
- Muscle wasting and/or slurred speech

Treatment options for nervous system vary because each condition causes different symptoms. In some cases, the condition can be cured or reversed with medical or surgical treatment. Unfortunately, many nervous system disorders have no cure – this is true for Alzheimer's disease, Huntington's disease, and Parkinson's disease. In cases that cannot be cured, medications or various other forms of therapy may help to manage symptoms and to slow the progression of the disease.

Chapter Two: Signs and Symptoms

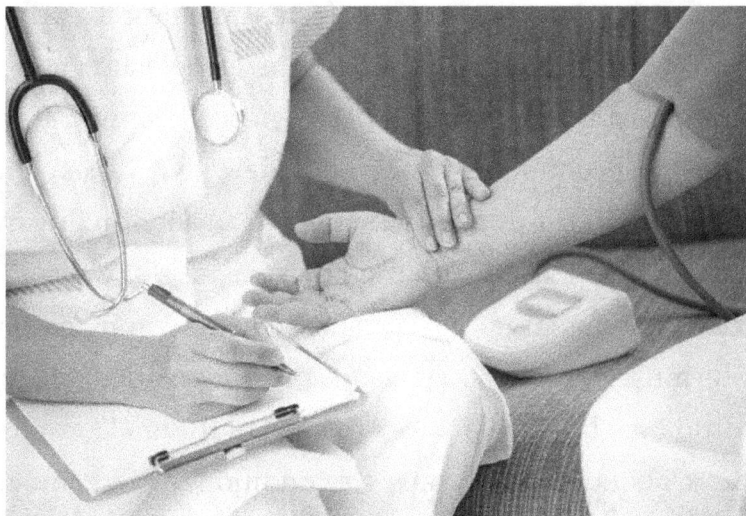

Now that you understand the basics about Charcot Marie Tooth disease and the history of the condition you may be curious about the different manifestations of the disease. In the next chapter you will learn the specifics about the different types of CMT but, in this chapter, you will receive some general information about the signs and symptoms of Charcot Marie Tooth disease as well as information regarding the progression of the disease. This information will help you to form a deeper understanding of CMT and how it affects the nervous system.

1. *Common Signs and Symptoms*

In most cases, symptoms of CMT manifest in early childhood or early adulthood. Some people, however, do not develop any symptoms until they reach their mid-thirties. The most common symptom people with CMT experience first is foot drop. Foot drop refers to an abnormality in a person's gait which is caused by weakness or damage to the common fibular nerve – it can also be caused by paralysis of the muscles in the lower leg. A person experiencing foot drop may be unable to flex the foot at the ankle or raise the toes. Foot drop often causes a condition called hammertoe in which the toes remain permanently curled.

As the disease progresses, many people with CMT experience a loss of sensation in their feet and legs as well as in the hands, wrists, and arms. Many people develop painful spasmodic muscular contractions and either high arched feet or flat arched feet. In many cases, both the sensory and the proprioceptive nerves in the feet and hands are damaged but the pain nerves are not. Thus, a person may lose sensory touch in the limb but might still feel pain. Continued use of the affected limb or hand can lead to additional symptoms like spasms, numbness, or painful cramping.

A few other symptoms that are frequently seen but often go unnoticed by the patient include involuntary teeth grinding and squinting. In some cases, the hearing, breathing, and vision of the patient can be affected as well. People with CMT often develop scoliosis, or abnormal curvature of the spine, which may lead to hunching and a loss of height. The hip sockets may also become malformed which can affect gait and mobility.

In some cases, gastrointestinal problems develop as a result of CMT. If the person suffers nerve damage, he or she may also have trouble chewing, swallowing or speaking. As muscles continue to waste and nerves degenerate, many people develop tremors or experience seizures. Prolonged stress and pregnancy have been known to exacerbate the symptoms of CMT, as can periods of prolonged immobility. All of these symptoms can lead to severe pain and muscular fatigue which can sometimes be mitigated with surgery, physical therapy, or assistive devices. When these therapies do not work to relieve pain, analgesic medications may be prescribed, depending on the severity.

As a result of skeletal malformations and muscle wasting, many people with CMT suffer frequent tripping and falling which can lead to serious injuries. Unfortunately, these injuries often cause a loss in mobility which can further exacerbate the other symptoms caused by CMT. Many people with CMT experience neuropathic pain which is described by the American Chronic Pain Association as, "a complex, chronic pain state that is usually accompanied by tissue injury... the nerve fibers themselves might be damaged, dysfunctional, or injured". As a result, the nerve fibers may send incorrect signals to various pain centers in the body which may or may not correlate to any injury or real stimulus.

2. Progression of the Disease

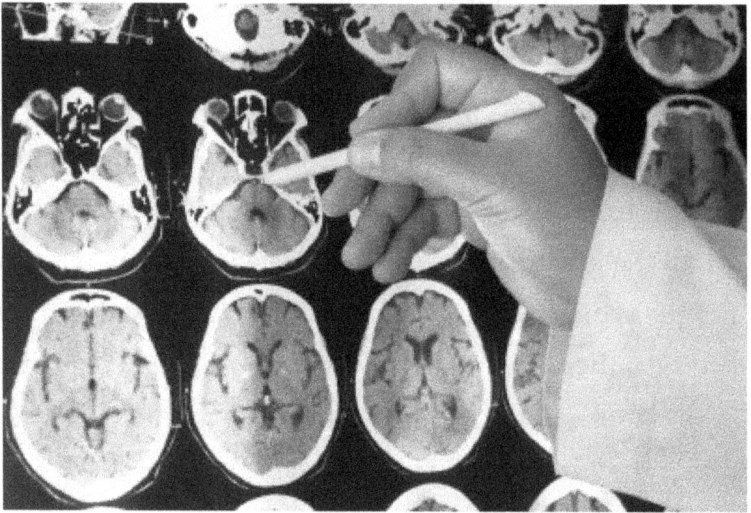

Although every case of Charcot Marie Tooth disease is different, most people experience a slowly progressing weakness and wasting of their distal muscles – the muscles that control the extremities. In most cases, the weakness starts in the feet and ankles, manifesting in the form of foot drop. This leads to trouble with walking and frequent tripping. As the weakness progresses, the patient makes greater attempts to compensate which can lead to the development of an abnormal gait.

While the early signs of CMT are easy to miss, many people become concerned and pay a visit to their doctor once they notice an increased frequency of trips and falls as well as other injuries related to the foot drop. To some degree, it is possible to compensate for the foot drop by wearing boots or shoes that support the ankles. Eventually, however, the problem becomes too severe and it must be dealt with in another way. Some people even end up wearing removable casts or leg braces around the foot and ankle to provide support.

People with late-stage CMT are likely to have lost so much muscle control that they require a wheelchair to get around. In many cases, people with late-stage CMT have also started to develop weakness in the hands and forearms – this may lead to trouble gripping things and making fine motor movements like buttoning clothes or turning a doorknob. Occupational therapy may be helpful in combating these developments.

Most cases of CMT only affect the muscles connected to the extremities but, in rare cases, the disease may cause increased weakness of the respiratory muscles. When this happens it can lead to life-threatening symptoms like shortness of breath. Respiratory problems caused by CMT can sometimes be treated with the use of a device that delivers air straight into the lungs.

In addition to physical symptoms like those discussed above, Charcot Marie Tooth disease can also lead to contractures or skeletal deformities. A contracture is a stiffened joint that occurs because the muscles around the joint have weakened. When some of the muscles around the joint are stronger than others, the stronger muscles will contract and pull on the joint which can cause the joint to shift into an abnormal position. For example, many people with CMT develop a shortened foot with a high arch because the muscles that lift the foot have weakened, causing the foot to curl downward. A small number of people with CMT may develop flat feet due to a different pattern of weakness in the foot muscles.

Not only can contractures affect the feet, but they can also affect the hands. As CMT worsens with time, contractures in the patient's hands can lead to the fingers becoming locked in a flexed position. Some people also develop scoliosis (abnormal curvature of the spine) or hip displacement. Regular stretching and physical therapy exercises can help to slow the progression of these symptoms and to prevent the development of contractures in CMT patients.

Chapter Three: Causes of the Disease

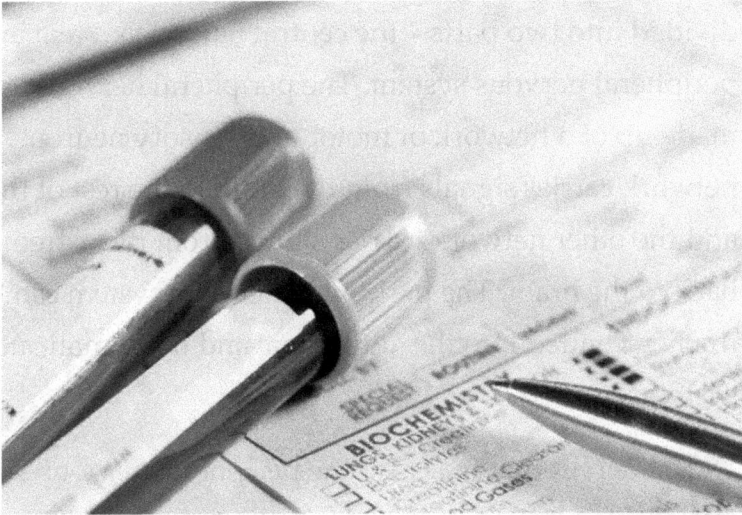

You have already learned that Charcot Marie Tooth disease is a condition affecting the peripheral nervous system, but you may be curious to learn exactly how it works. In this chapter you will receive some background information about the causes of CMT disease as well as information regarding inheritance of the disease. Additionally, you will receive an overview of the different types and subtypes of Charcot Marie Tooth disease including the symptoms and effects of each.

1. What Causes Charcot Marie Tooth Disease?

As you may already know, the human nervous system is divided into two parts – the central nervous system and the peripheral nervous system. The peripheral nervous system is made up of a network of motor and sensory neurons. One network carries signals from the brain to the rest of the body and the other network carries signals from the extremities back to the brain. The peripheral nervous system can be further divided into the autonomic and the somatic nervous systems.

The nerves that make up the peripheral nervous system (called peripheral nerves) are similar to electrical wires – they have an inner core (called the axon) which is protected by the myelin sheath (acts as insulation). When the myelin sheath on any peripheral nerve becomes damaged, peripheral nerve impulses may slow down – if the axon is damaged, the speed of the connection may remain the same but the strength of the signal is weakened. These two things are the core dividers between type 1 and type 2 for Charcot Marie Tooth disease.

The causes of CMT are genetic and most forms involve damage to the axon or demyelination. Genetic defects in the genes for certain proteins that affect the axons or the myelin sheath are the driving force behind CMT. Because CMT is the result of genetic mutation, there are as many kinds of CMT as there are related genes – there are about 80 different genes that have been linked to CMT so far and more are likely to be discovered.

In some cases, Charcot Marie Tooth disease presents in a similar way to various types of acquired neuropathy – this is a kind of nerve damage caused by chemical exposure, diabetes, drug use, or immunological abnormalities. In reality, however, CMT is a hereditary condition and it is not contagious. Because it is passed down from one generation to another, CMT is also sometimes called hereditary motor and sensory neuropathy, or HMSN. There are three ways that CMT can be inherited:

- **X-Linked** – This type of inheritance occurs when the mutated gene is located on the X chromosome. X-linked diseases tend to affect men more often than women because women have two X chromosome – if one copy is normal it might be able to compensate adequately for the defective copy. An X-linked disease cannot be passed on from father to son.

- **Autosomal Dominant** – Autosomal inheritance occurs on some other type of chromosome, not the

X or Y – for this reason, autosomal diseases affect men and women equally. An autosomal dominant inheritance occurs when a single copy of the mutated gene is enough to cause the disease – if a person inherits a mutated gene from their parent, both of them will have the disease.

- **Autosomal Recessive** – In this type of inheritance, two copies of the mutate gene are necessary to cause the disease. The person would receive one copy of the mutated gene from each parent and, in most cases, neither of the parents have actually developed the disease.

When CMT is inherited through autosomal dominant inheritance, it is easy to trace the disease on the patient's family tree. Both X-linked and autosomal recessive inheritance, however, are harder to track. This is because one or both parents may not actually have the disease but they are carriers of it. In addition to these three types of inheritance, there is one more way that CMT can occur. In rare cases, a spontaneous mutation may occur during conception which can cause CMT. In cases like this, the child can then grow up to genetically pass the disease on to his or her children.

The risk for passing on CMT from one generation to the next depends largely on the type of CMT. The age at which a person who is genetically predisposed to the disease varies as well. People with type 1 generally start to develop symptoms in late childhood or early adolescence while people with type 2 typically present with symptoms later in life – around early adulthood or middle age. The rate of progression for the disease varies from one type to another, though most cases progress very slowly.

2. Types of Charcot Marie Tooth Disease

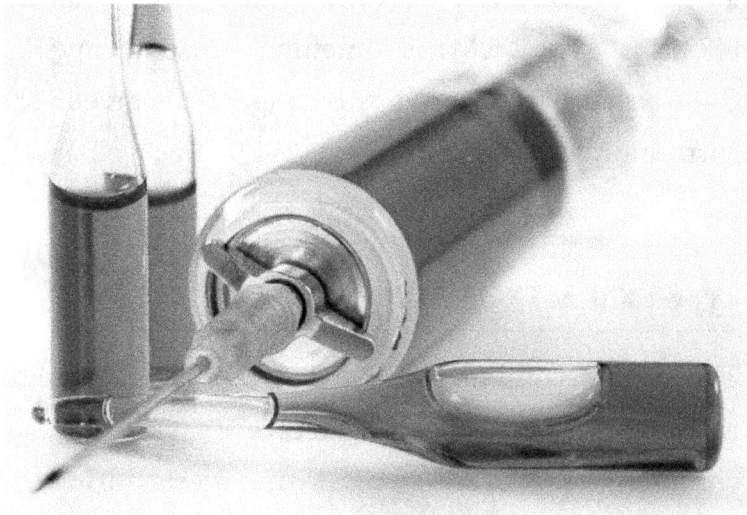

There are two main types of Charcot Marie Tooth disease – type 1 and type 2. Within each of these types, however, there are several subtypes. There are also more severe versions of the disease which have been labeled type 3 and type 4. In this section you will receive an overview of the different types and subtypes for CMT.

Type 1 (CMT 1)

The most common type of CMT is type 1 – it accounts for about two-thirds of CMT cases and it is inherited with an autosomal dominant pattern. The primary symptoms associated with type 1 include muscle atrophy and weakness and loss of sensation, typically in the feet, legs, hands, and forearms. Type 1 CMT is sometimes caused demyelinating CMT because it is caused by damage to the myelin sheath surrounding the nerves.

Type 1 X (CMTX or CMT 1X)

This is the second most common type of CMT, accounting for between 10% and 16% of all cases that are found on the X chromosome. This type typically manifests during childhood or adolescence and it is inherited with an X-linked pattern. CMTX presents symptoms similar to type 1 and type 2 but it usually affects males more severely than it affects females. A male with CMTX can pass it to his daughter, but not to his son. A woman with CMTX has a 50% chance of passing it to any of her children.

Type 2 (CMT 2)

This type of CMT is caused by axonopathy – or damage to the axon of the nerves which impacts their response. CMT 2 presents in a similar way to CMT 1, though it can be either autosomal dominant or autosomal recessive. Type 2 is sometimes associated with other conditions like restless legs syndrome – this condition can be treated.

Type 3 (CMT 3)

Also known as Dejerine-Sottas Syndrome (DSS), type 3 CMT is characterized by a thinning of the myelin around the affected nerve. This type is very severe and it is often seen in disabled patients who develop the disease during infancy (or before age 3). The name for this condition was determined before any of the genetic causes for CMT were identified, so the name DSS is used more frequently than CMT type 3. This type of CMT can be inherited with either an autosomal dominant or recessive pattern.

Type 4 (CMT 4)

This type of CMT is fairly rare and it is inherited in an autosomal recessive pattern. CMT 4 may vary in severity from one case to another and, in many cases, the patient exhibits symptoms in other parts of the body such as loss of hearing or vision. Because type 4 usually has a very early onset it is sometimes called Severe, Early-Onset CMT. When children have CMT 4, the often display delayed motor development and low muscle tone.

Subtypes of Charcot Marie Tooth Disease

Now that you have a basic understanding of the four main types of CMT you will be able to grasp the details for each of the subtypes. There are multiple subtypes for Type 1, Type 2 and Type 3 CMT but not for Type 3, Dejerine-Sottas Syndrome. Below you will find an overview of the subtypes for each type of CMT:

CMT Type 1

Type 1A – This is the most common subtype for CMT, comprising nearly two-thirds of all cases of CMT type 1. Type 1A is caused by a duplication of the PMP22 gene on the 17th chromosome. Rather than just having two copies of the gene, the patient has three copies – two on one chromosome and one on the other. People with CMT 1A usually develop high arches and hammertoe with varying degrees of hand weakness and balance problems.

Type 1B – This type of CMT is caused by mutations of the peripheral myelin protein (MPZ) gene. Type 1B varies in severity from one case to another with early onset being much more severe than later onset, in most cases. People with CMT 1B usually have slow nerve conduction velocities which can lead to developmental delays.

Type 1C – CMT Type 1C is caused by various disease-causes mutations in the LITAF gene. This form of CMT is very rare, affecting less than 1% of people with diagnosed CMT. The presentation of Type 1C is similar to Type 1A and it usually sets in between the ages of 10 and 30, presenting with weakness in the feet and hands then progressing to muscle atrophy and sensory loss.

Type 1D – This type of CMT is caused by mutations of the EGR2 gene on the 10th chromosome – this is the gene responsible for early growth response. Like Type 1C, Type

1D is very rare and only accounts for about 1% of all CMT cases. Most patients with CMT Type 1D show symptoms before the age of 10 – these may include delayed motor development and slow nerve conduction velocities.

Type 1E – This type of CMT is caused by mutations in the PMP22 gene. The severity of this type varies, but people with Type 1E tend to exhibit earlier onset and more serious symptoms than people with Type 1A. In many cases, children with Type 1E present by the age of 2 with symptoms of delayed walking. Many people with Type 1E end up needing ambulation aids such as walkers and wheelchairs later in life.

Type 1F – This is an autosomal dominant form of the disease and it is very rare. Type 1F is caused by a defect in the neurofilament light chain protein located on the 8th chromosome.

Type 1X – Also known as CMTX, this subtype is the second most common form of CMT. Type 1X is caused by a gap in the junction between the beta 1 protein and connexin 32 on the X chromosome. This type of CMT usually manifests in childhood or adolescence, affecting males more severely than it affects females.

CMT Type 2

Type 2A – This type of CMT is caused by a defect in the MFN2 gene on chromosome 1p36. The defect occurs in the fusion of the mitochondria.

Type 2B – Type 2B Charcot Marie Tooth disease is caused by a defect in the RAB7 protein located on the 3rd chromosome. This type is characterized by significant problems with ulceration and it presents with largely sensory symptoms. In fact, some researchers believe that Type 2B is nothing more than sensory neuropathy, not actually a subtype of CMT.

Type 2C – This type of CMT is incredibly rare and it has been linked to the 12th chromosome. Type 2C has also been linked to patients with vocal cord or diaphragm paresis in addition to other CMT symptoms.

Type 2D – This form of CMT is caused by mutations in the glycyl RNA synthetase gene on chromosome 7p14. This type of CMT can be very confusing because some patients exhibit sensorimotor neuropathies while others only show motor symptoms.

Type 2E – Little is known about Type 2E but it has been linked to chromosome 8p21 in connection to mutations of the neurofilament light gene.

Type 2O – This type of CMT is a rare kind of axonal neuropathy and it is inherited in an autosomal dominant pattern. Type 2O is caused by mutation of the dynein cytoplasmic 1 heavy chain 1 gene, or CYNC1H1 located on chromosome 14. This type usually manifests with motor weakness rather than sensory impairment.

CMT Type 4

Type 4A – This type of CMT is caused by a mutation in the GDAP 1 protein on the 8th chromosome. The first cases of this type of CMT were identified in a Tunisian family that was highly inbred. The onset for this type is usually around age 2 and it manifests in the form of delayed developmental milestones like walking and sitting. Most patients with Type 4A become wheelchair-bound by the age of ten.

Type 4B – This form of CMT is caused by a genetic defect in the 11th chromosome. Type 4B usually presents by the age of 3 years and it usually causes both distal and proximal weakness.

Type 4C – New research suggest that Type 4C is the most common autosomal recessive form of the CMT disease – this means that the patient must have two copies of the mutated gene in order to develop the disease. This type is caused by a mutation of the SH3TC2 gene on the 5th chromosome. Type 4C usually presents with early-onset deformities of the spine and slowly progressing neuropathy.

Type 4D – This type of CMT is linked to the 8th chromosome and it was first discovered in a Gypsy population. This form is inherited with an autosomal recessive pattern and it causes severely reduced nerve conduction. Other symptoms typically include distal weakness, sensory loss, muscle atrophy, and hand or foot deformities. Deafness usually develops by the age of 30.

Type 4F – This form of CMT is very severe and it has only been observed in a large Lebanese family who were found to have mutations in the TRX gene located on the 19th chromosome. Nerve biopsies revealed onion bulb formations as well as slow nerve conduction.

Type 4J – This type of CMT is caused by mutations in the FIG4 gene on the 6th chromosome. This form of CMT is still very rare and it was only identified for the first time in 2007. Type 4J varies in terms of onset and symptoms and it has an autosomal recessive pattern of inheritance. This type usually causes slow nerve conductions caused by changes in the myelin sheath around the affected nerve.

Chapter Four: Diagnosis and Prognosis

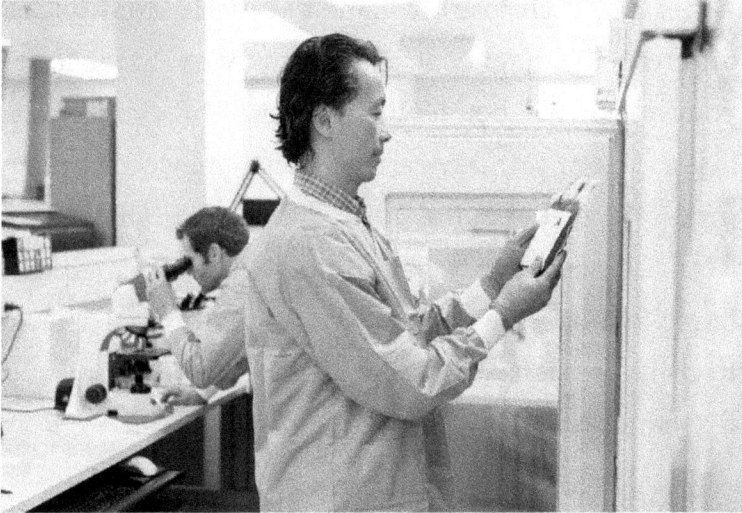

Unfortunately, some of the symptoms associated with Charcot Marie Tooth disease have also been correlated with other neurological disorders – this makes achieving an accurate diagnosis somewhat tricky. Still, there are certain tests and diagnostic techniques physicians can use to correctly diagnose CMT. In this chapter you will learn the basics about how a doctor goes about diagnosing a person with Charcot Marie Tooth disease – you will also learn about the prognosis for this condition.

1. Diagnosis of the Disease

Because each case of Charcot Marie Tooth disease is different, the diagnostic process can vary. In most cases, your doctor will begin with a detailed medical and family history. Your primary care physician may be able to get this process started, but it is best to have the exam performed by a trained neurologist. In addition to taking a medical and family history, the doctor will also perform an array of tests to check for signs of muscle weakness or foot deformities like hammertoe, high arches, and foot drop.

To test your muscle strength and/or sensory loss, your doctor might have you try walking on your heels – he may also ask you to press your leg against his hand as an opposing force. To check for sensory loss, the doctor may test your deep tendon reflexes – if they are reduced or absent, it is likely a sign of CMT. While performing these tests, the doctor will ask you questions about other common CMT symptoms to support the diagnosis.

Another test that is commonly used to diagnose CMT is called an electromyogram (EMG) or a nerve conduction velocity (NCV) test. This is a type of electrodiagnostic testing which can be used to measure the speed and strength of the electrical signals travelling through your peripheral nervous system. A delayed nervous response may be indicative of demyelination which is associated with Type 1 CMT. Reduced response is usually a sign of axonopathy which is correlated with Type 2 CMT. This test can also help to gauge the strength of electrical signals in your arm and leg muscles.

In some cases, a nerve biopsy may be taken to confirm a diagnosis and to identify the type of CMT the person has. This is usually necessary in cases where the patient doesn't have a complete family history or his symptoms are very mild or very severe. A neurologist can study the patient's DNA by taking a blood sample to check for duplication of certain genes – this can also help to identify the type of CMT the person has.

2. Prognosis for the Disease

Unfortunately, there is no cure for Charcot Marie Tooth disease. The condition is almost always inherited, which means that it is not contagious. It is also worth noting that the disease usually progresses very slowly so it is unlikely to have a negative effect on the patient's lifespan. The disease can, however, affect the patient's mobility. There are a number of different treatment options available for different types of CMT which can help the patient manage his or her symptoms.

Chapter Five: Treatment Options

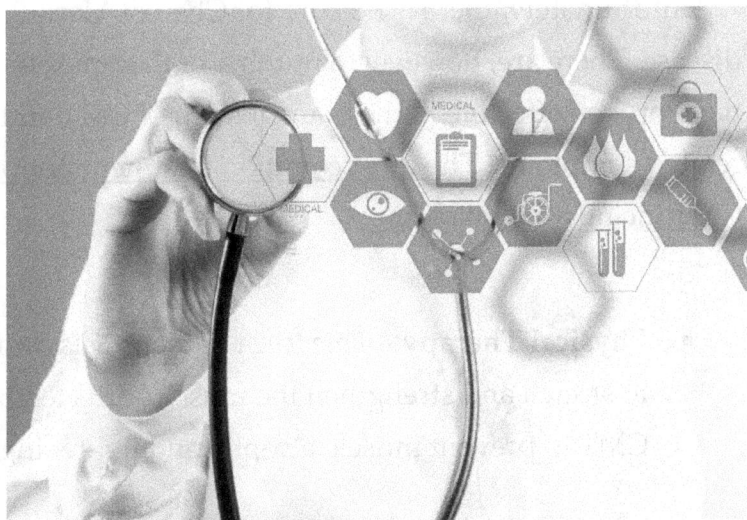

For the most part, Charcot Marie Tooth disease is a slowly progressing disease and the symptoms can be managed with a variety of therapies. Different forms of CMT require different treatment options, some of which can be paired to ensure more thorough management of the condition. In this chapter you will learn about the various treatment options available to CMT patients as well as the different types of the disease they are typically used to treat. You will learn the specifics about dietary support options for CMT in the next chapter.

1. Overview of Treatment Options

Unfortunately, there is no cure for Charcot Marie Tooth disease. There are, however, a number of therapies which have proven effective in the management of CMT and its related symptoms. <u>The most common treatment options for CMT include the following</u>:

- **Physical Therapy** – This form of therapy is designed to stretch and strengthen the muscles affected by CMT to prevent muscle atrophy and tightening.

- **Occupational Therapy** – This type of therapy is similar to physical therapy but it is designed to help patients develop and strengthen the motor skills necessary to complete normal daily activities.

- **Orthopedic Devices** – Braces, splints, and other orthopedic devices may be necessary for people with CMT who have experienced muscle atrophy or changes in mobility.

- **Surgery** – This type of therapy is usually performed to correct physical deformities or as a treatment for injuries related to CMT.

- **Medication** – Certain drugs can be prescribed to help manage and reduce the symptoms related to various forms of CMT.

The type of treatment recommended will vary depending on the type and severity of your Charcot Marie Tooth disease. Many people who have CMT engage in regular physical or occupational therapy not only to manage their symptoms but to slow their progression as well. Periods of immobility are particularly dangerous for CMT patients because it can lead to loss of muscle control and sensitivity that can be hard to regain. In the following pages you will learn more about each of the different CMT treatment options in greater detail.

2. Physical and Occupational Therapy

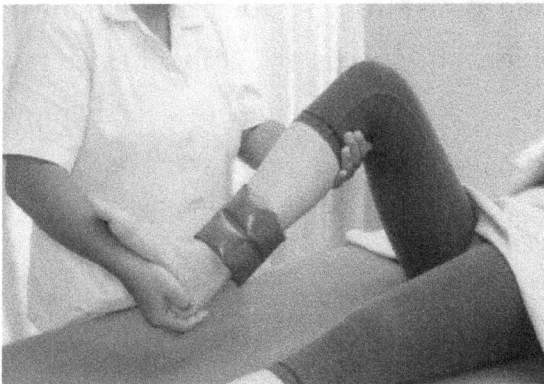

Physical therapy involves performing specific exercises to help stretch and strengthen the muscles. Occupational therapy, on the other hand, involves practicing or re-learning how to perform daily tasks such as buttoning a shirt, writing, or handling silverware. Because muscle wasting and nerve deterioration are such common symptoms of peripheral neuropathy, most people diagnosed with CMT undergo physical and/or occupational therapy at some point.

Many people with Charcot Marie Tooth disease see a physical or occupational therapist two or three times per week. To maximize the benefits of these therapies, it is best to start them as early as possible – before the problem becomes advanced. For example, if you start regular physical therapy before you loss a significant amount of muscle mass in your legs, it can actually help to keep your bones and joints strong so you can avoid most of the loss. Occupational therapy is primarily directed toward weakness in the hands and arms, while physical therapy is usually directed toward the legs and lower body.

3. Braces and Orthopedic Devices

In many cases, Charcot Marie Tooth disease leads to certain foot deformities which may require the use of special braces or orthopedic devices. For example, an ankle-foot orthosis (AFO) is very commonly used by CMT patients. An AFO is a type of removable cast that fits tightly around the patient's foot and ankle. Early versions of the AFO were cumbersome and heavy, made primarily of metal. Today, however, they are made of lightweight plastic and can be worn under pants. Splints are another type of orthopedic device frequently used by people who develop foot contractures.

There is some debate regarding the efficacy of night splinting. Some doctors suggest that splinting the legs overnight can help to reduce mobility problems while others say that it has no effect in increasing range of motion in the ankle. For the most part, braces and orthopedic devices are only used by CMT patients to provide support during motion and during the execution of everyday tasks. Canes and walkers may also help to provide support and to increase mobility for CMT patients.

4. Surgical Procedures

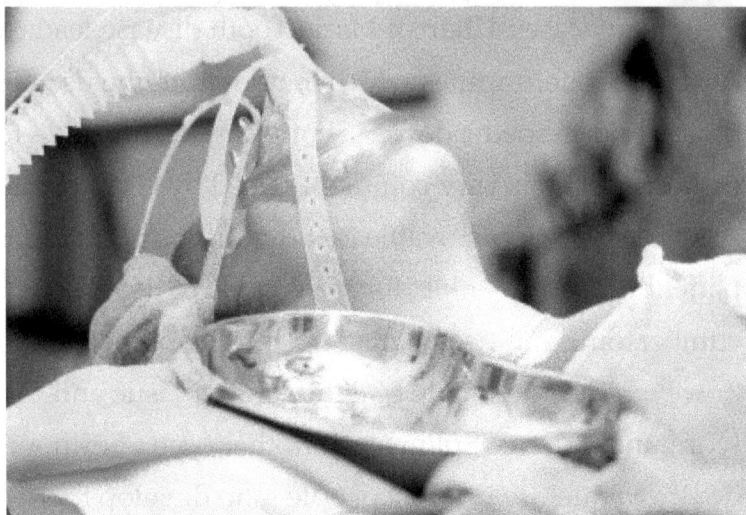

Approximately 50% of Charcot Marie Tooth disease patients develop some kind of foot or ankle problem. The deformity known as cavovarus is the most common – it is a kind of flexible deformity that forms during childhood or adolescence and it usually becomes resolved by adulthood. Some of the most common surgical procedures performed on CMT patients include:

- **Soft-Tissue Surgeries** – These may include tendon transfers, tendon releases, and plantar fasciotomies.

- **Triple Arthrodesis** –This procedure involves a fusion of the talocalcaneal, calcanocuboid, and talonavicular joints and it is only performed in severe cases as a method of pain relief.

- **Osteotomies** – This procedure may be performed on the metatarsal, calcaneal, tarsometatarsal, or tarsal bones.

Surgery can be performed to correct physical deformities caused by CMT or to repair injuries. It cannot, however, be used to improve muscle weakness or any loss of sensation the patient may have.

5. Medical Management

Depending on the type of Charcot Marie Tooth disease you have, certain medications may be prescribed to help you manage symptoms. Unfortunately, some prescription drugs have been known to actually exacerbate the symptoms of CMT and may even lead to acquired neuropathy. This is why it is extremely important that you consult your physician before taking any new drugs and follow the dosage instructions very carefully. You may even want to do some of your own research before starting a new drug, checking for side effects – especially those that mention words like neuropathy, neuropathic pain, paresthesia, or peripheral nerve damage.

When it comes to managing CMT-related pain, it is important to realize that there are different types of pain. Musculoskeletal pain related to joint problems or muscle soreness may respond to nonsteroidal anti-inflammatory drugs (NSAIDs) or simply to acetaminophen. Neuropathic pain, on the other hand, may be better managed with antiepileptic drugs or tricyclic antidepressants. Again, always make sure you follow your doctor's recommendations when starting a new medication and follow dosing instructions carefully.

6. Additional Treatments and Therapies

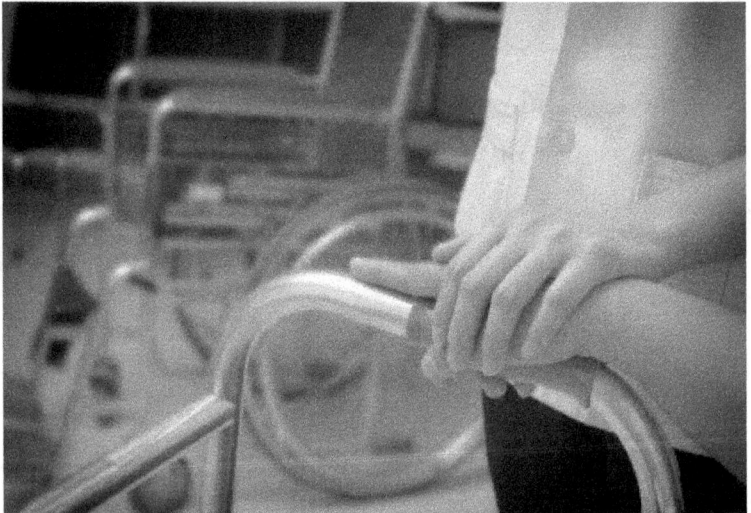

Thanks to recent developments in genetic research, there are some new gene therapies for Charcot Marie Tooth disease in the works. Certain gene therapies, for example, might be targeted toward the specific genetic defect responsible for the disease while others are likely to be focused on repairing the damage caused by those defective genes. Some of these therapies are currently being tested in animal trials – it will still be some time before they can be tested on humans.

In addition to the therapies described in the previous pages, there are also some home remedies and lifestyle changes you can incorporate to manage your CMT. For example, stretching regularly at home can help you to maintain and improve your range of motion – it may also help you to improve balance, coordination, and flexibility. In some cases, regular stretching can even help to prevent CMT-related joint deformities that often result from muscle atrophy or uneven pulling on the joint.

Not only can regular stretching help to manage your CMT, but regular exercise in general is always a good thing. It is best to stick to low-impact exercises like biking and swimming because they put less stress on your joints and muscles which could be weakened by the disease. Regular use of your muscles and joints can help to increase mobility and flexibility.

If you have problems with stability, you may want to try walking with a cane or a walker. Making sure your home is properly lit will help you to avoid injuries caused by stumbling or falling. You should also pay close attention to your feet – keep your nails trimmed to avoid ingrown toenails and infections but be sure to cut them straight across, not into the nailbed. Always wear shoes that fit you well and try to choose shoes that provide additional support at the ankle. If you have already developed hammertoe or other foot deformities, you may need to have special shoes made.

Chapter Six: Dietary Support Options

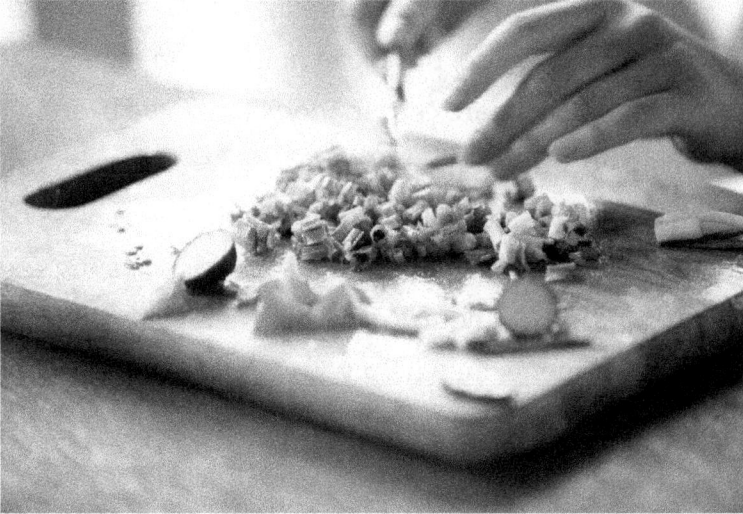

After reading the last chapter you should have a good idea what treatment options for Charcot Marie Tooth disease look like. Again, the best treatment for CMT will vary depending on the type and progression of the disease. Many people with CMT can experience further relief from symptoms by making changes to their diet. Certain foods have been associated with improved muscle recovery which can help CMT patients. In this chapter you will receive an overview of foods that aid muscle recover and receive some simple recipes using these ingredients.

1. Supplements for Peripheral Neuropathy

Making changes to your diet may not cure your Charcot Marie Tooth disease, but it can help you to manage your symptoms. There are certain foods that have been identified as being able to aid in muscle recovery – this is an important part of CMT therapy. The following nutrients have been identified as potential treatments not for CMT in particular but for peripheral neuropathy in general – <u>these nutrients and supplements may help you to manage your condition more effectively</u>:

- **L-Carnitine** – This nutrient is produced in the body through biosynthesis of two amino acids, lysine and methionine. There is some research to suggest that l-carnitine may be an effective treatment for peripheral neuropathy, though more research is required.

- **Biotin** – Also known as Vitamin B7, biotin is a water-soluble vitamin which is essential for certain enzymes to work in the body. Again, more research is needed but biotin has been suggested as a potential treatment for various forms of peripheral neuropathy.

- **Folate** – Folic acid, or folate, is another type of water-soluble B vitamin (B9). This vitamin has been suggested as a means of improving symptoms related to peripheral neuropathy. Folate is the naturally-occurring form of this vitamin – folic acid is the synthetic form.

- **Vitamin B12** – A deficiency in Vitamin B12 has been shown to worsen the symptoms of peripheral neuropathy, especially in diabetics.

- **Alpha-Lipoic Acid** – A powerful antioxidant, alpha-lipoic acid has been used for years in Europe as a treatment for peripheral neuropathy.

- **Curcumin** – The results of several research studies suggest that supplementation with curcumin may help to prevent the development of neuropathic pain.

- **Vitamin B1** – Also known as benfotiomine, Vitamin B1 is a fat-soluble vitamin that may help to reduce neuropathic pain and to improve nerve conduction velocity.

Some of the nutrients or supplements listed above must be taken in synthetic form but some of them can be found in certain foods. Below you will find a list of food sources that contain some of the nutrients listed on the previous page. These are the ingredients that are used in the recipes provided later in this chapter.

Foods to Improve Peripheral Neuropathy

- Asparagus
- Artichokes
- Avocado
- Beans
- Beef
- Beets
- Brewer's Yeast
- Broccoli
- Brussels Sprouts
- Chickpeas
- Cottage Cheese
- Curry Powder
- Eggs
- Fish
- Legumes
- Lentils
- Milk
- Nuts
- Nutritional Yeast
- Oatmeal
- Oranges
- Organ Meats
- Papaya
- Pork
- Poultry
- Red Meat
- Rice Bran
- Romaine Lettuce
- Seeds
- Spinach
- Soy Milk
- Tempeh
- Tomatoes
- Turmeric
- Wheat Germ
- Whole-Grain Cereal
- Whole Wheat Bread
- Yams

- Yogurt (low-fat)

2.) *Foods to Avoid for Peripheral Neuropathy*

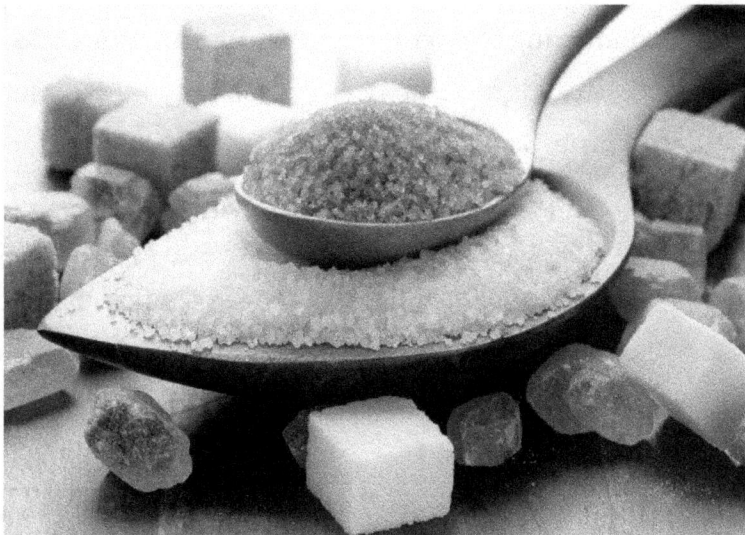

Just as there are certain foods and supplements which can help to manage the symptoms of peripheral neuropathy, so are there foods that may aggravate your symptoms. <u>The following foods are best avoided by people with CMT and other forms of neuropathy</u>:

- **Refined Grains** – Things like all-purpose flour and other high-glycemic grains can have a serious impact on your blood sugar. Controlling blood sugar is an important aspect of preventing neuropathy, especially neuropathy that is associated with diabetes.

- **Gluten** – Foods containing gluten can be especially damaging for people with gluten allergies and celiac disease. It has also been correlated with worsening symptoms of neuropathy.

- **Added Sugar** – Refined sugars add calories to food without increasing the nutritional value. Nutritional deficiencies have been shown to worsen symptoms of neuropathy.

- **Saturated Fats** – Full-fat dairy products and fatty cuts of meat are loaded with saturated fats which can cause inflammation and worsening of neuropathic symptoms.

3. Recipes for Muscle Support and Recovery

The following recipes are made with many of the ingredients listed in Section 1 of this chapter. These foods many help you to reduce the symptoms associated with your peripheral neuropathy. Just be sure to consult your physician before you make any significant changes to your diet, even if it is to help with your CMT.

Recipes Included in this Chapter:

Eggs Baked in Avocado

Cinnamon Apple Overnight Oats

Tomato Basil Omelet

Homemade Whole-Grain Muesli

Curried Chickpea Burgers

Balsamic Avocado Spinach Salad

Coconut Vegetable Curry

Vegan Cream of Broccoli Soup

Warm Quinoa and Veggie Salad

Roasted Beet Soup

Rosemary Roasted Chicken and Veggies

Herb-Crusted Pork Tenderloin

Easy Beef and Vegetable Stir-Fry

Avocado Chocolate Mousse

Blueberry Yogurt Parfait

Eggs Baked in Avocado
Servings: 4

Ingredients:

- 2 large ripe avocadoes
- 4 large eggs
- 1/3 cup reduced-fat shredded cheese
- Salt and pepper to taste
- 1 green onion, sliced thin

Instructions:

1. Preheat the oven to 425°F and line a small baking dish with foil.
2. Cut the avocados in half, removing the pit.
3. Scoop out 2 to 3 tablespoons from the middle of each avocado then place the halves cut-side up in the baking dish.
4. Crack one egg into the middle of each avocado half.
5. Sprinkle with cheese and season with salt and pepper.
6. Bake for 16 to 20 minutes until the egg is cooked to the desired level.
7. Season garnished with sliced green onion.

Cinnamon Apple Overnight Oats

Servings: 4

Ingredients:

- 2 cups unsweetened soy milk
- 2 cups whole-grain oats, uncooked
- 1 cup low-fat yogurt, plain
- 1 cup unsweetened applesauce
- 1 to 1 ½ teaspoons ground cinnamon

Instructions:

1. Combine the soy milk and oats in a large mixing bowl.
2. Stir in the yogurt, applesauce, and cinnamon.
3. Mix the ingredients until thoroughly combined.
4. Spoon the mixture into four glass jars and cover with the lids.
5. Refrigerate the jars overnight and serve in the morning.

Tomato Basil Omelet

Servings: 1

Ingredients:

- 2 teaspoons olive oil
- 1 medium vine-ripened tomato, cored and chopped
- ¼ cup diced yellow onion
- 1 clove minced garlic
- 2 large eggs, beaten well
- Salt and pepper to taste
- 1 tablespoon fresh chopped basil

Instructions:

1. Heat 1 teaspoon of oil in a small skillet over medium heat.
2. Add the tomato, onion, and garlic then cook for 2 to 3 minutes until the onion is softened.
3. Spoon the vegetables off into a bowl and reheat the skillet with the remaining oil.
4. Pour the beaten eggs into the skillet and season with salt and pepper.
5. Let the eggs cook for 1 to 2 minutes until they start to set.
6. Spoon the vegetable mixture over half the omelet and top with the chopped basil.

7. Let the egg cook until almost set then fold the empty half of the omelet over the fillings.
8. Cook for 30 to 60 seconds until the eggs are done then slide onto a plate to serve.

Homemade Whole-Grain Muesli

Servings: 10 to 12

Ingredients:

- 4 cups old-fashioned oats, uncooked
- 1 cup sliced almonds
- ½ cup chopped pecans
- 1 ½ cups shredded unsweetened coconut
- 2 to 3 tablespoons raw honey
- 2 tablespoons coconut oil, melted
- 1 ½ teaspoons vanilla extract
- 1 teaspoon ground cinnamon
- ½ teaspoon salt
- 1 cup seedless raisins

Instructions:

1. Preheat the oven to 350°F and line a rimmed baking sheet with parchment.
2. Toss together your oats, almonds, pecans, and coconut in a mixing bowl.
3. Stir in the honey, coconut oil and vanilla along with the salt and cinnamon.

4. Spread the mixture in the baking sheet and bake for 12 to 16 minutes until toasted, stirring once halfway through.
5. Allow the muesli to cool then toss in the raisins.
6. Store in an airtight container and serve in bowls drizzled with soy milk.

Curried Chickpea Burgers

Servings: 8

Ingredients:

- ½ cup old-fashioned oats, uncooked
- 2 medium carrots, peeled and grated
- 1 tablespoon coconut oil
- 1 (15-ounce) can chickpeas, rinsed and drained
- ¼ cup toasted sunflower seeds
- 1 ½ teaspoons curry powder
- ¼ teaspoon paprika
- ¼ teaspoon turmeric
- Salt and pepper to taste
- 8 whole-grain sandwich buns, toasted

Instructions:

1. Preheat the oven to 375°F and line a baking sheet with parchment.
2. Combine your oats, carrots and coconut oil in a food processor and blend until well combined.

3. Pulse in the chickpeas about ½ cup at a time, leaving some of them mostly whole.
4. Add the sunflower seeds, curry powder, paprika, and turmeric then season with salt and pepper to taste.
5. Pulse a few more times to combine then shape the mixture into eight even-sized patties by hand.
6. Place the patties on the baking sheet and bake for 20 minutes until heated through.
7. Serve the burgers hot on toasted whole-grain sandwich buns.

Balsamic Avocado Spinach Salad

Servings: 4

Ingredients:

- 6 to 8 cups fresh chopped spinach
- 1 cup thinly sliced cucumber
- 1 medium red bell pepper, cored and sliced thin
- 1 cup cherry tomatoes, halved
- ¼ cup extra-virgin olive oil
- 3 tablespoons balsamic vinegar
- 1 teaspoon Dijon mustard
- 1 teaspoon honey
- 1 clove minced garlic
- 1 ripe avocado, pitted and sliced thin
- 2 green onions, sliced thin

Instructions:

1. Toss together the spinach, cucumber, bell peppers and tomatoes in a salad bowl.
2. In a separate small bowl, whisk together the olive oil, balsamic vinegar, mustard, honey and garlic.
3. Toss the salad with the dressing then divide evenly among four salad plates.
4. Top each salad with a few slices of avocado.
5. Garnish with sliced green onion to serve.

Coconut Vegetable Curry

Servings: 6 to 8

Ingredients:

- 1 tablespoon olive oil
- 1 medium yellow onion, chopped
- 1 cup fresh chopped broccoli florets
- 1 cup fresh chopped cauliflower florets
- ½ cup sliced carrots
- 1 tablespoon fresh minced garlic
- 1 tablespoon fresh grated ginger
- 1 cup low-sodium vegetable broth
- 2 (14-ounce) cans coconut milk
- 1 tablespoon curry powder
- 1/8 teaspoon cayenne (optional)
- 1 cup fresh sugar snap peas

- ¼ cup fresh diced tomatoes

Instructions:

1. Heat the olive oil in a large saucepan over medium heat.
2. Add the onion, broccoli, cauliflower and carrot.
3. Stir in the garlic and ginger then sauté for 4 to 6 minutes until the vegetables are just tender.
4. Add the vegetable broth, coconut milk, curry powder, and cayenne.
5. Bring the mixture to a boil then reduce heat and simmer for 10 to 15 minutes.
6. Stir in the snap peas and tomatoes then cook for 2 minutes more before serving hot over steamed brown rice.

Vegan Cream of Broccoli Soup

Servings: 6

Ingredients:

- 1 ½ tablespoons coconut oil
- 1 small yellow onion, chopped
- Salt and pepper to taste
- 1 medium stalk celery, sliced thin
- 1 teaspoon minced garlic
- 4 cups low-sodium vegetable broth
- ½ lbs. Yukon gold potatoes, peeled and chopped

- 4 cups fresh chopped broccoli florets
- ½ cup unsweetened soy milk

Instructions:

1. Heat the oil in a large saucepan over medium heat.
2. Stir in the onion and season with salt and pepper to taste.
3. Cook for 6 to 8 minutes until browned then stir in the celery and garlic.
4. Sauté the ingredients for 5 minutes then stir in the vegetable broth and potatoes.
5. Bring to a boil then reduce heat and simmer for 12 to 15 minutes until the potatoes are tender.
6. Stir in the broccoli then cover and cook for 5 minutes until it is bright green.
7. Remove from heat and puree the soup using an immersion blender.
8. Whisk in the soymilk and adjust seasonings to taste then serve hot.

Warm Quinoa and Veggie Salad

Servings: 6 to 8

Ingredients:

- 1 cup uncooked quinoa, rinsed well
- 1 cup water
- 1 teaspoon coconut oil

- 1 small yellow onion, chopped
- 1 medium red bell pepper, cored and chopped
- 1 cup diced zucchini
- 4 cups fresh chopped romaine lettuce
- ¼ cup extra virgin olive oil
- 1 tablespoon red wine vinegar
- 1 teaspoon fresh lemon juice salt and pepper to taste

Instructions:

1. Stir together the quinoa and water in a medium saucepan.
2. Bring the mixture to boil then reduce heat and simmer, covered, for 15 to 20 minutes until the quinoa absorbs the water.
3. Remove the quinoa from heat and set aside to cool slightly.
4. Heat the coconut oil in a large skillet over medium heat.
5. Add the onion, peppers and zucchini and sauté for 4 to 6 minutes until tender.
6. Place the chopped lettuce in a serving bowl.
7. Whisk together the red wine vinegar and lemon juice then season with salt and pepper.
8. Drizzle in the olive oil while whisking.
9. Toss the cooked vegetables and the quinoa in with the lettuce then toss with the dressing to serve.

Roasted Beet Soup

Servings: 4

Ingredients:

- 1 lbs. medium-sized beets, scrubbed clean
- 1 tablespoon coconut oil
- 1 medium yellow onion, chopped
- 1 medium leek, chopped (white and light green part only)
- 2 small stalks celery, sliced thin
- 4 cups water
- ½ teaspoon fresh chopped thyme
- ½ teaspoon fresh ground ginger
- Salt and pepper to taste

Instructions:

1. Preheat the oven to 350°F and wrap your beets in foil.
2. Place the foil-wrapped beets in the oven and roast for about 1 hour until fork-tender.
3. Cool the beets then peel them and chop coarsely.
4. Heat the oil in a large saucepan over medium-high heat.
5. Stir in the onion, leek, and celery then cook for 8 to 10 minutes until browned.
6. Add the roasted beets along with the water and seasonings.

7. Bring the mixture to a boil then reduce heat and simmer for 20 to 25 minutes until the vegetables are very tender.
8. Remove from heat and puree the soup using an immersion blender.
9. Drizzle with soy milk or top with a dollop of yogurt to serve.

Rosemary Roasted Chicken and Veggies

Servings: 6 to 8

Ingredients:

- 1 tablespoon olive oil
- 8 to 10 bone-in chicken drumsticks
- Salt and pepper to taste
- 2 large carrots, peeled and sliced
- 2 medium yams, peeled and chopped
- 1 large yellow onion, chopped
- 1 cup chopped broccoli florets
- 1 cup chopped cauliflower florets
- ½ cup low-sodium chicken broth
- 1 to 2 tablespoons dried rosemary

Instructions:

1. Preheat the oven to 400°F and grease a 9x13-inch glass baking dish with cooking spray.
2. Heat the oil in a large skillet over medium heat.

3. Season the chicken with salt and pepper to taste then add to the skillet.
4. Cook for 2 to 3 minutes on each side until browned.
5. Toss together the vegetables in the baking dish then place the chicken on top, skin-side down.
6. Drizzle with chicken broth and sprinkle with rosemary.
7. Roast for 30 minutes then turn the chicken and roast for another 25 to 30 minutes until the juices run clear.
8. Let the dish cool for 10 minutes before serving.

Herb-Crusted Pork Tenderloin

Servings: 6

Ingredients:

- 2 tablespoons extra-virgin olive oil
- 1 tablespoon fresh minced garlic
- 2 teaspoons fresh chopped rosemary
- 1 teaspoon dried thyme
- 1 teaspoon dried basil
- Salt and pepper to taste

Instructions:

1. Preheat the oven to 475°F.
2. Combine the olive oil, garlic, rosemary, basil, and thyme in a small bowl and stir well then season with salt and pepper to taste.

3. Rub the mixture into the pork tenderloin on all sides then place it on a roasting pan.
4. Roast for about 30 minutes then reduce the oven temperature to 425°F.
5. Let the pork roast for another 50 to 60 minutes until the internal temperature reads 155°F.
6. Remove the tenderloin to a cutting board and let rest 15 to 20 minutes before slicing.

Easy Beef and Vegetable Stir-Fry

Servings: 4 to 6

Ingredients:

- 2 tablespoons olive oil
- 1 lbs. lean beef sirloin, sliced thin
- Salt and pepper to taste
- 2 cups fresh chopped broccoli florets
- 1 medium red pepper, cored and chopped
- 1 small yellow onion, chopped
- ½ cup sliced carrots
- 2 tablespoons hoisin sauce
- 1 tablespoon low-sodium soy sauce
- 1 tablespoon water
- 1 clove minced garlic
- 1 teaspoon cornstarch
- ½ teaspoon toasted sesame oil
- ¼ teaspoon ground ginger

Instructions:

1. Heat the oil in a large skillet over medium-high heat.
2. Season the beef with salt and pepper to taste then add it to the skillet.
3. Cook for 1 to 2 minutes on each side until just browned then move the beef to the sides of the skillet.
4. Add the vegetables and stir-fry for 2 to 3 minutes.
5. Whisk together the remaining ingredients and pour into the skillet.
6. Stir-fry for another 2 to 3 minutes until the mixture is heated through and the sauce is thickened.
7. Serve hot over steamed brown rice or quinoa.

Avocado Chocolate Mousse

Servings: 4 to 6

Ingredients:

- ½ cup dark chocolate chips
- 4 medium ripe avocadoes, pitted and chopped
- ½ cup raw honey
- ½ cup unsweetened cocoa powder
- 6 tablespoons milk
- 2 teaspoons vanilla extract

Instructions:

1. Melt the chocolate chips in a double boiler on low.

2. Once the chocolate is melted, remove from heat and stir smooth.
3. Combine the melted chocolate and avocado in a food processor.
4. Add the honey, cocoa powder, milk and vanilla extract.
5. Blend until smooth and well combined then spoon into dessert cups.
6. Chill for at least 4 hours before serving.

Blueberry Yogurt Parfait

Servings: 4

Ingredients:

- 2 cups old-fashioned oats
- 2 tablespoons raw honey
- ½ teaspoon ground cinnamon
- 2 cups low-fat yogurt, plain
- 2 cups fresh blueberries

Instructions:

1. Preheat the oven to 350°F and line a rimmed baking sheet with parchment.
2. Toss the oats with the honey and cinnamon then spread evenly on the baking sheet.
3. Bake for 15 to 20 minutes, stirring once, until toasted and browned.

4. Spoon about ¼ cup of oats into the bottom of each of four parfait glasses.

5. Top each with ½ cup yogurt and ¼ cup blueberries.

6. Repeat the layers, using the remaining oats and yogurt then topping off with the rest of the blueberries.

Chapter Seven: Research

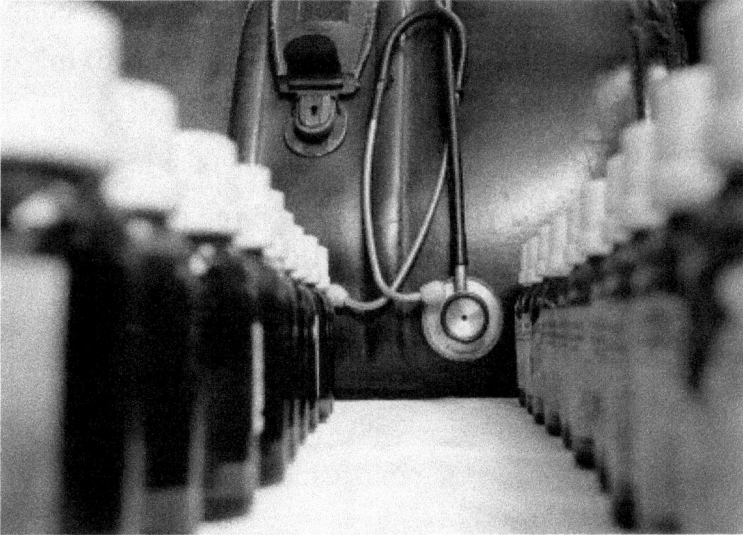

As you should thoroughly understand by now, Charcot Marie Tooth disease is a complex condition that comes in many forms. Great leaps and bounds have been made regarding CMT research in the past two decades but there is still a great deal more to learn. In this chapter you will learn about the kind of research that is currently being conducted regarding CMT. You will also receive some information about clinical trials that are currently or will soon be conducted.

1. What Research is Being Conducted?

Charcot Marie Tooth disease was first described in 1886 but there is still a great deal to be learned about this disease. Only within the past few decades has genetic research advanced enough to enable researchers to identify and study the various subtypes for this condition. In fact, the genetic causes for CMT were only discovered in 1991. About a decade later, scientists had identified ten genes linked to CMT as well as evidence suggesting several other genetic correlations. These same developments in genetic research have also improved genetic testing options for Charcot Marie Tooth disease.

One of the main areas of CMT research currently being conducted is in regard to the underlying causes of the disease. Researchers are studying the processes that are involved in the destruction of axons and the thinning of myelin so that they can create therapies to counteract these problems. More specifically, researchers are studying not only what defects cause CMT, but how those defects actually cause the disease.

In addition to researching the underlying causes of Charcot Marie Tooth disease, scientists are also working to develop new therapies. The first step in this process is to develop a reliable research model so these new therapies can be tested accurately. Current research studies regarding the development for CMT therapies are being conducted with both mouse and fly models. Scientists are also working on models made from stem cells harvested from patients with CMT.

There are two main types of CMT therapy currently in development – drug therapy and gene therapy. Researchers are trying to develop therapies that are specific to certain subtypes of the disease, hoping to identify a treatment that will target the specific genetic defect responsible for the disease. In one example, researchers are using non-toxic viruses as a method of delivery. In other studies, researchers are trying to find a way to block the production by the mutated gene or to replace it entirely. For drug therapy, researchers are studying applications that might help reduce or reverse axonopathy and demyelination.

The Charcot-Marie-Tooth Association

One of the biggest names in CMT research is the Charcot-Marie-Tooth Association (CMTA). This organization was originally founded in 1983 as the National Foundation for Peroneal Muscular Atrophy (NFPMA). The group was founded by Dr. Howard Shapiro, a CMT patient himself, in an attempt to increase awareness of the disease within the medical community. In addition to raising awareness for CMT, Dr. Shapiro also hoped to provide support for patients and families dealing with the disease that, at that point, was still poorly understood.

Within a few years of starting the foundation, Dr. Shapiro had raised enough funds to organize the Second International Research Conference which was held at Arden House on the campus of Columbia University. After the conference, research efforts and journal publications related to CMT increased drastically. Over the next decade, a large number of significant breakthroughs in CMT research occurred. These included:

- Correlation of CMT Type 1A with chromosome 17
- Identification of the Peripheral Myelin Protein (PMP22) nerve
- The cause of Hereditary Neuropathy with Liability to Pressure Palsies (HNPP)
- Mutation of the MPZ gene linked to CMT Type 1B
- Cause of CMT Type 1X by point mutations in connexin 32 gene

Another of Dr. Shapiro's great achievements was the establishment of the North American CMT Database. This database allows researchers to have access to a record of families identified by the type of CMT they carry – this helps give doctors a better understanding of the clinical symptoms associated with particular subtypes. The database also helps to increase awareness about the severity and the progression of CMT.

Today, the CMTA's vision is to achieve, "A world without CMT". The foundation is dedicated to supporting the development of new drug therapies, improving the quality of life for CMT patients, and finding a cure for the disease. The CMTA is led by a board of directors made up of 18 of the world's leading CMT experts and researchers. The foundation currently supports more than 30,000 patients and families through the database.

2. Clinical Trials for CMT Disease

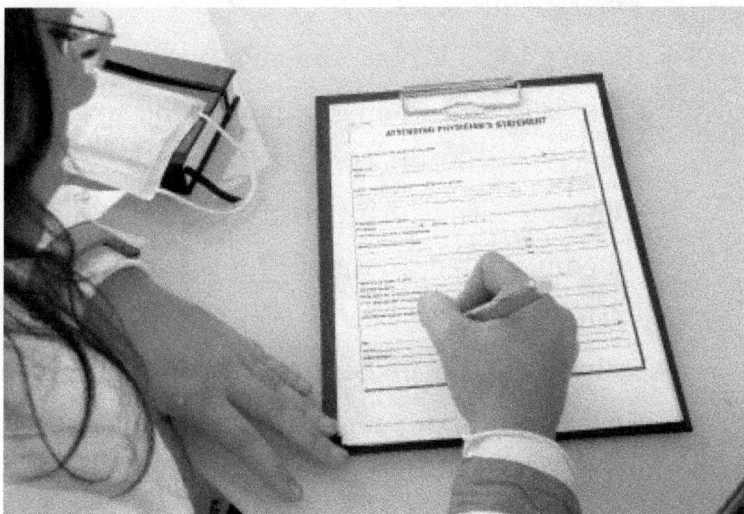

When new therapies are tested on animals or insects it is referred to as a study or simply research. If the therapy is tested on humans, however, it is referred to as a clinical trial. A clinical trial is carefully regulated and designed to follow a specific order of steps to divide the study into different phases. These phases are:

- **Observational** – This phase involves testing the biomedical or health outcomes of the therapy in order to further understand the course of the disease.
- **Phase 0** – This phase involves testing the distribution of the new drug throughout the body at a very low dose – a dose that is below the therapeutic level.
- **Phase 1** – This phase involves testing the safety of the drug on a small group of people in order to determine the effective dosage.
- **Phase 2** – This phase involves testing the drug on a medium-sized group of people to determine its safety.
- **Phase 3** – This phase involves testing the drug on a larger group of people to determine its safety and to monitor side effects.

- **Phase 4** - This phase involves studying the drug after it has been marketed in order to further understand its benefits and side effects in correlation with long-term use.

One of the leaders in CMT clinical trials is the Muscular Dystrophy Association (MDA). This organization supports studies designed to understand the disease and for the development of new therapies. As an example, one clinical trial is currently testing the benefits of strength training in CMT patients.

Some of the other clinical trials that will be conducted in the future are listed by name on the following page:

- Development of CMT Pediatric Scale for Children with CMT
- Correlation Between Clinical and Electrophysiological Phenotypes in a Population of Patients with Neuropathy CMT Type 1A
- Driving Ability in Patients with CMT Type 1A
- Genetics of CMT –Modifiers of CMT1A, New Causes of CMT2
- Natural History Evaluation of CMT Types CMT1B, CMT2A, CMT4A, CMT4C, and Others
- Evaluation of the Analgesic Efficiency of the Transcutaneous Neurostimulation in the Charcot

Syndrome Marie Tooth on the Pains of the Lower Limbs

- Study of Electrical Impedance Myography (EIM) in ALS
- Genetics of Pediatric-Onset Motor Neuron and Neuromuscular Diseases
- Treadmill, Stretching and Proprioceptive Exercise Rehabilitation Program for CMT Neuropathy Type 1A (CMT1A)

Chapter Eight: Frequently Asked Questions

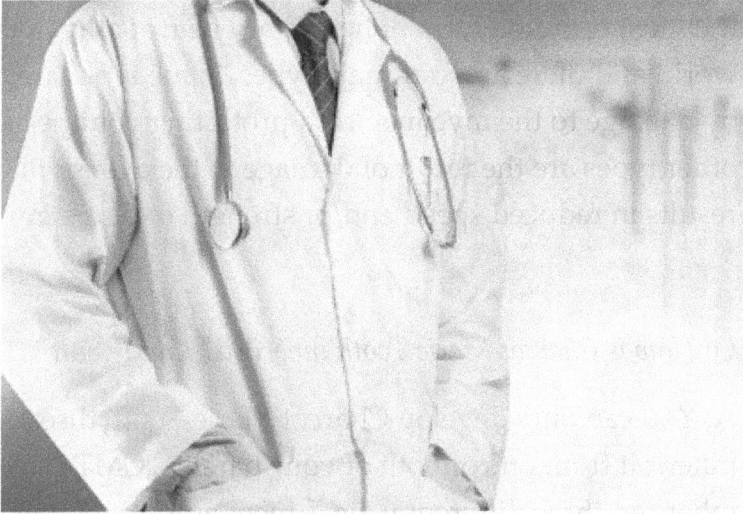

In reading this book you have received a wealth of information about Charcot Marie Tooth disease including its causes, presentation, and treatment options. Even after reading this book, however, you may find that you still have questions – that is where this chapter comes into play. In this chapter you will receive a list of frequently asked questions about Charcot Marie Tooth disease to help you gain a better understanding of this condition and its management.

Q: *What is the cause of CMT?*

A: Charcot Marie Tooth disease comes in many forms, but it is generally caused by some kind of genetic defect. CMT is the most common form of hereditary neuropathy in the world and there are four main types. Some types are caused by damage to the myelin sheath protecting your nerves and other types are the result of damage to the axons which results in reduced speed and/or strength of nerve impulses.

Q: *How is Charcot Marie Tooth inherited? Can I get it?*

A: You can only develop Charcot Marie Tooth disease if you inherit it from one or both of your parents. CMT can be inherited three different ways – in an autosomal dominant, autosomal recessive, or X-linked pattern. It is possible for someone to develop CMT if neither of their parents have it, but their parents must be carriers.

Q: *How can I find out what kind of CMT I have?*

A: Thanks to advances in modern genetic research, it is now possible to identify the specific genetic defect responsible for causing CMT. Your neurologist will perform a series of tests in addition to taking a detailed history and physical exam to determine which type of CMT you have. Once that has been determined your doctor will make specific recommendations for treatment.

Q: *How can I expect my CMT to progress over time?*

A: For the most part, CMT is a slowly progressing disease but you can expect it to get worse with time. It is difficult to project the course of progression because each case is different. If you have one of the more common forms of the disease you may be able to reference case studies to get an idea what the progression for your own CMT may look like.

Q: What exactly does CMT do to the body?

A: CMT is a type of peripheral neuropathy which means it affects the nerve signals traveling between your brain and your extremities. In many cases, CMT causes severe muscle atrophy and neuropathic pain – it can also lead to physical deformities, usually of the feet.

Q: *Is it common for CMT to be diagnosed or treated inaccurately?*

A: There is always a possibility for misdiagnosis, especially because there are so many different types and presentations for CMT. Unfortunately, neuromuscular diseases are misdiagnosed with some regularity – patients may be told that their symptoms are psychosomatic. In some cases it can take multiple examinations and several specialists to make a correct diagnosis or to choose the right treatment. Taking the wrong medication can lead to serious problems, so always be careful about starting a new drug.

Q: *How will my CMT be treated?*

A: Treatment options for CMT vary depending on the type and progression of the disease. Starting physical and/or occupational therapy as early as possible will help to reduce muscle weakness and to address problems with mobility. In some cases, you may also need orthopedic devices or surgery to manage or correct physical deformities. Certain medications have also been used to relieve CMT symptoms but there are some medications which can actually make things worse so you need to be very careful.

Conclusion

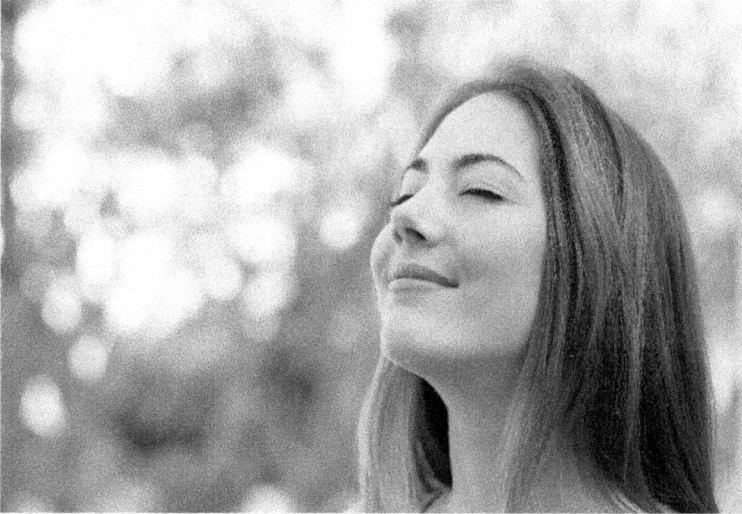

By now you should have a thorough understanding of Charcot Marie Tooth disease. CMT is by no means an easy disorder to have or to deal with, but there are some good treatment options available. Because treatment options vary from one form of CMT to another, it is important that you see your physician to run the various tests required to identify which kind of CMT you have and which treatment option is best for you.

Although there is no cure for Charcot Marie Tooth disease, important research is still being conducted and more is learned about this disease each and every year. The key to managing your CMT is to learn as much about the condition as you can. The more you know about the underlying cause for your CMT, the better equipped you will be to handle the symptoms and to manage your condition. By making changes to your diet and partnering with your physician on medical, surgical, and physical therapies you can get your CMT under control and experience the best quality of life possible.

Index

A

B

E

F

G

H

I

J

L

l-carnitine	59
legs	13, 15, 22, 34, 35, 51, 52

M

malformation	9
management	47, 48, 99
manifestation	13
medications	20, 23, 55, 102
men	30, 31
mobility	23, 46, 48, 52, 57, 102, 112
motor	6, 26, 29, 30, 35, 37, 39, 40, 48
multiple sclerosis	19

muscle 6, 15, 19, 23, 26, 34, 35, 37, 41, 44, 48, 49, 50, 51, 54, 55, 57, 58, 59, 101, 102

muscle loss	6
muscles	9, 13, 15, 22, 23, 25, 26, 27, 45, 48, 50, 57
Muscular Dystrophy Association	97, 112, 113, 114, 115
mutations	7, 13, 36, 37, 39, 41, 94
myelin sheath	29, 34, 42, 100
myelopathy	15

N

nerve 9, 12, 22, 23, 24, 29, 30, 35, 37, 41, 42, 44, 45, 50, 55, 60, 94, 100, 101

nerve impulses	10, 29, 100
nervous disorders	2, 11, 18, 19, 116
nervous system	6, 11, 12, 17, 18, 19, 21, 28, 29, 44

S

T

V

W

X

References

"Carnitine." National Institutes of Health.
   <https://ods.od.nih.gov/factsheets/Carnitine-
   HealthProfessional/>

"Charcot-Marie-Tooth (CMT)." Yale School of Medicine.
   <https://medicine.yale.edu/neurology/patients/neuromus
   cular/cmt.aspx>

"Charcot-Marie-Tooth Disease." Mayo Clinic.
   <http://www.mayoclinic.org/diseases-conditions/
   charcot-marie-tooth-disease/basics/definition/con-
   20029920>

"Charcot-Marie-Tooth Disease (CMT)." Muscular Dystrophy
   Association. <https://www.mda.org/
   disease/charcot-marie-tooth/overview>

"Charcot Marie Tooth Disease." Patient.info.
   <http://patient.info/doctor/charcot-marie-tooth-disease>

"Charcot Marie Tooth Disease Information and Facts."
   Disabled World. <http://www.disabled-
   world.com/disability/types/mobility/charcot-marie-tooth-
   disease.php>

"Clinical Trials." Muscular Dystrophy Association.
   <https://www.mda.org/disease/charcot-marie-
   tooth/clinical-trials>

"CMTA Mission and History." Charcot-Marie-Tooth
    Association. <http://www.cmtausa.org/about-us/cmta-
    mission-and-history/>

"Facts About Charcot-Marie-Tooth Disease & Related
    Diseases." Muscular Dystrophy Association.
    <https://www.mda.org/sites/default/files/publications/Fa
    cts_CMT_P-180_0.pdf>

"Food Sources of Folate." Dietitians of Canada.
    <http://www.dietitians.ca/Your-Health/Nutrition-A-
    Z/Vitamins/Food-Sources-of-Folate.aspx>

Kedlaya, Divakara. "Charcot-Marie-Tooth Disease."
    Medscape. <http://emedicine.medscape.com/
    article/1232386-overview>

"Learning About Charcot Marie Tooth Disease." National
    Human Genome Research Institute.
    <https://www.genome.gov/11009201>

"Nervous System Problems – Topic Overview." WebMD.
    <http://www.webmd.com/brain/tc/nervous-system-
    problems-topic-overview>

"Neuropathic Pain." American Chronic Pain Association.
    <http://www.theacpa.org/condition/neuropathic-pain>

"Nutrition." The Foundation for Peripheral Neuropathy.
    <https://www.foundationforpn.org/livingwithperipheral
    neuropathy/neuropathynutrition/>

"Nutrition for Neuropathy." Diabetes Self-Management. <http://www.diabetesselfmanagement.com/blog/nutritio n-for-neuropathy/>

"Organization of the Nervous System." RCN.com. <http://users.rcn.com/jkimball.ma.ultranet/BiologyPages/ P/PNS.html>

"Overview of Nervous System Disorders." Johns Hopkins Medicine. <http://www.hopkinsmedicine.org/ healthlibrary/conditions/nervous_system_disorders/over view_of_nervous_system_disorders_85,P00799/>

"Research." Muscular Dystrophy Association. <https://www.mda.org/disease/charcot-marie- tooth/research>

"Supplement Treatments for Neuropathy." Dr. Whitaker. <http://www.drwhitaker.com/supplement-treatments- for-neuropathy/>

"Types and Causes." Charcot-Marie-Tooth Association. <http://www.cmtausa.org/understanding-cmt/types-and- causes/>

"Types of CMT." Muscular Dystrophy Association. <https://www.mda.org/disease/charcot-marie- tooth/types-cmt>

"Vitamin B1 for Energy." Dr. Weil. <http://www.drweil.com/drw/u/ART02760/vitamin-b1>

"What is CMT?" Charcot-Marie-Tooth Association. <http://www.cmtausa.org/understanding-cmt/what-is-cmt/>

Additional Titles Available...

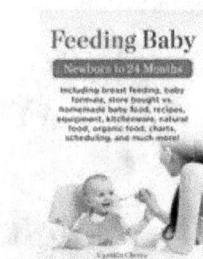

Feeding Baby
Cynthia Cherry
978-1941070000

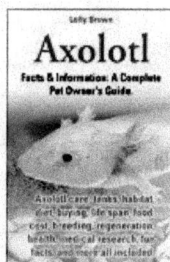

Axolotl
Lolly Brown
978-0989658430

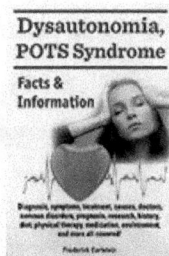

Dysautonomia, POTS
Syndrome
Frederick Earlstein
978-0989658485

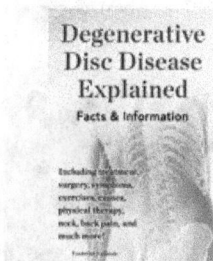

Degenerative Disc
Disease Explained
Frederick Earlstein
978-0989658485

Additional Titles Available…

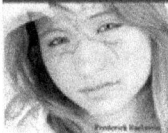

Sinusitis, Hay Fever,
Allergic Rhinitis Explained
Frederick Earlstein
978-1941070024

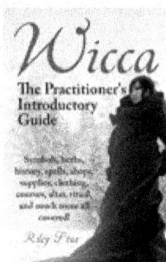

Wicca
Riley Star
978-1941070130

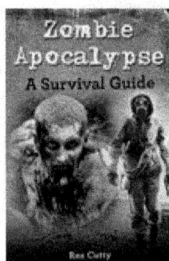

Zombie Apocalypse
Rex Cutty
978-1941070154

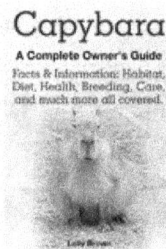

Capybara
Lolly Brown
978-1941070062

Additional Titles Available...

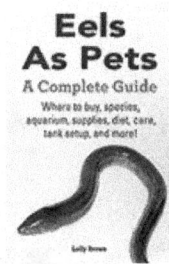

Eels As Pets
Lolly Brown
978-1941070167

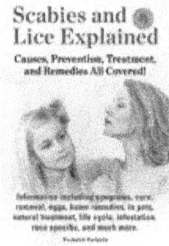

Scabies and Lice Explained
Frederick Earlstein
978-1941070017

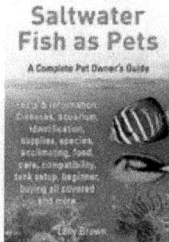

Saltwater Fish As Pets
Lolly Brown
978-0989658461

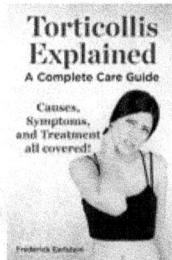

Torticollis Explained
Frederick Earlstein
978-1941070055

Additional Titles Available…

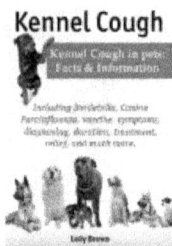

Kennel Cough
Lolly Brown
978-0989658409

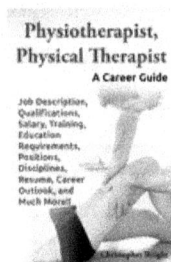

Physiotherapist, Physical
Therapist
Christopher Wright
978-0989658492

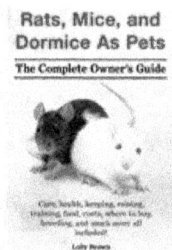

Rats, Mice, and Dormice
As Pets
Lolly Brown
978-1941070079

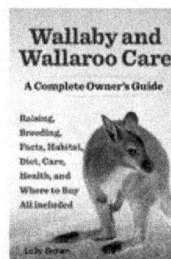

Wallaby and Wallaroo Care
Lolly Brown
978-1941070031

Additional Titles Available…

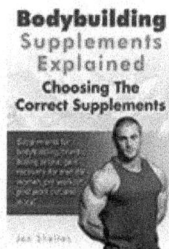

Bodybuilding Supplements
Explained
Jon Shelton
978-1941070239

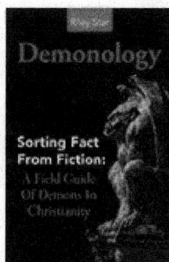

Demonology
Riley Star
978-19401070314

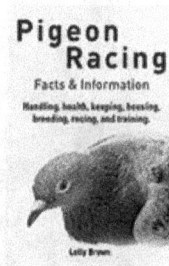

Pigeon Racing
Lolly Brown
978-1941070307

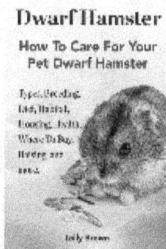

Dwarf Hamster
Lolly Brown
978-1941070390

Additional Titles Available…

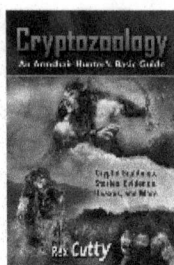

Cryptozoology
Rex Cutty
978-1941070406

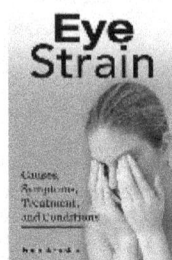

Eye Strain
Frederick Earlstein
978-1941070369

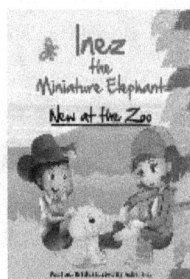

Inez The Miniature Elephant
Asher Ray
978-1941070353

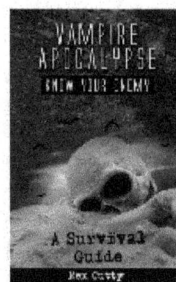

Vampire Apocalypse
Rex Cutty
978-1941070321

www.ingramcontent.com/pod-product-compliance
Lightning Source LLC
Chambersburg PA
CBHW050535280326
41933CB00011B/1600